Meet the Follicles

by Ciara Foskin

978-1-917728-26-3

© 2025 Ciara Foskin

All rights reserved. No part of this book may be reproduced, stored in a retrieval system, or transmitted by any means, electronic, mechanical, photocopying, recording or otherwise without written permission from the author. Author views are their own.

This publication is for your personal use only and not meant to reflect any medical advice. If you have any medical concerns please consult the relevant professional.

Cover design and illustrations © Dave Comiskey

Published in Ireland by Orla Kelly Publishing.
Orla Kelly Publishing
27 Kilbrody,
Mount Oval,
Rochestown,
Cork,
Ireland.

I am made and remade continually.
Different people draw different words from me.
Every encounter is a version of myself being rewritten.
There is no final self, only motion.

Virginia Woolf
The Waves (1931)

Dedicated to my mother, Anne, and my Aunt Phyllis, two very special women whom I miss very much.

Introduction

There it is— a hint of light reflects onto my hair, finally catching my short strands.

A shine that has been almost a year in the making. Newly shorn, my follicles have grown back into short, thick locks.

Inside, I'm nearly dancing.

Just like frogspawn turns to tadpoles and then frogs, my body, mind, and soul have endured an enormous transformation. My worldview has shifted, been fine-tuned, and I am forever changed.

—

No two breast cancers are the same. I've learnt this since my diagnosis in February 2024. While there are, of course, common elements to what I've come to see as an incredibly complex illness, how it affects our lives, bodies, and psyches differs greatly.

Some of us will question if we are to blame, combing back through our lives searching for why we are now in this hell. We talk to other women diagnosed with breast cancer to help us understand our experience and get emotional support. We look for commonalities to bond us together at a time when we need people like never before.

Before I got cancer, I was a happy, 46-year-old parent of one with a zest for life and fairly active. Life was good. I worked from home, enjoyed time with my daughter, Saibh, now 11 years old, and spent my free time swimming with friends in The Guillamene, Tramore, Co. Waterford.

Then, in November 2022, my mother passed away unexpectedly at the age of 74. She had heart issues for a few years, but we weren't prepared for her to go when she did. It was a massive shock and a trauma for me and my family. Little did I know what was still to come.

In late 2023, I found a small hard lump in my breast and thought it was just a cyst since I was prone to them. This time, though, it was different. Thankfully, I got it checked when I did, or things could have ended a lot worse for me.

On February 8th, 2024, I was diagnosed with Triple Negative Breast Cancer (TNBC) Stage 2B—one of the rarer, more aggressive breast cancers. I'd never heard of it, and the more I learned about it, the more frightened I became. I remember asking my surgeon at University Hospital Waterford (UHW) whether this kind was better or worse than others. His reply? "This isn't the one you'd want." Each appointment—from diagnosis through to my first chemotherapy session—brought more information, more bad news. I also had genetic testing, which showed I carried a CHEK2 gene mutation, increasing my chance of getting breast cancer by up to 40%.

Long story short, the treatment was brutal. I was prescribed eight sessions of chemotherapy, double major surgery (bilateral mastectomy and reconstruction), recovery, three weeks of radiotherapy, and then eight cycles of oral chemotherapy. 'Prescribed' being the operative word here. Chemo hammered me so hard that I only managed three sessions before it had to be stopped. Surgery was moved up to late June 2024, and I spent the summer recovering. It was rough. Throw in total hair loss, a crushing breakup (a blessing in disguise, to be honest), and the realisation that cancer doesn't just test you—it reveals the true nature of everyone around you. Thankfully, the majority of people in my life are pretty wonderful.

Radiotherapy was the easiest part for me. Don't get me wrong, going to Whitfield for 15 consecutive days to have your chest area zapped while you daren't move during it is highly unpleasant. But compared to chemo and surgery, it was less brutal. I swanned in, chatted with the regulars every afternoon while my daughter, Saibh, started into fourth class. I was fatigued but managed well overall. Then came the oral chemo, which floored me. My body couldn't tolerate the ten daily tablets. I got so unwell that it was stopped.

Since then, I've been recovering, though cancer-related fatigue, medical tests, and appointments are constant companions. Life feels more precious now, and I savour everything—big or small. Cancer has changed me, inside and out.

Post-cancer
- I've a much lower tolerance level for noise which can stress me. Emotional and physical trauma have taken their toll

- Negative people drain me. I prefer being around those who appreciate life and bring positivity

- Your mental health is as important as your physical health. I found that if I was feeling down, I couldn't cope as well with the physical discomfort. Talking to a professional is crucial

- I'm more laid-back, relish every day, and live in the present

- My time is now for people who are kind, bring joy, and laughter

- Physically, I'm still sore in places and tire easily. I can't walk long distances, I get winded quickly, and just don't have the energy I used to. This is really challenging for me

- My hair, once long, is short now. Sporting a bald head was so hard, but now I've grown to love my short crop

- I've learned that you can plan for the future, but in an instant, everything can change. We can plan all we want, but nothing is guaranteed

I've seen how resilient I am and how my inner drive has carried me through cancer. As I'm a naturally positive and social person, this has helped me endure the harder days. Kindness, support, love, and laughs matter so much, and of course, dipping in the sea!

2025 has brought light and positive moments. I'm proud to be an Ambassador for Triple Negative Breast Cancer with the Marie Keating Foundation. I've shared my story on KCLR radio and with The Irish Examiner, and have met incredible people along the way.

Last year, I found writing poetry as a way to help make sense of my new world after diagnosis. My normality was gone—I was craving my old body and life pre-cancer, and I was full of grief. Writing gave me the creative outlet I needed to express my feelings and thoughts while allowing me to frame the multitude of things I'd endured.

I'd written poems before—my first back in 2014. Thankfully, I kept the notebooks; publishing them is something I never expected to do, but lo and behold, cancer made me do it. With that said, there are many other pieces of writing in this book about other areas of my life over the past ten years, not about cancer.

I also want to share with you a few dos and don'ts when interacting with people with cancer. From my own experience and from talking to a psychologist who has counselled thousands of cancer patients, it's important to know how to be around someone with cancer.

These words, born from grief and transformation, are deeply personal, and they're for anyone navigating similar paths.

I don't promise you a happy read, but this is my story, through my words.

Do's and Don'ts for Cancer Support

So, I'd like to talk a little about the things people say to you when you're going through cancer. A person's words can give you real comfort, or have the complete opposite effect. There are times when you bite your tongue and inside, you're just so taken aback by the lack of awareness and understanding of someone saying the 'wrong' thing to you. It can cause hurt and distress and make you feel more alone in your illness.

Looking Beyond Appearances
Often, people don't know what to say—especially if you look outwardly healthy during your illness. Looks can be deceiving. Speaking from my experience, I could appear completely fine on the outside while dealing with intense fatigue, physical weakness, and internal and external scars. It's disheartening when, as you try to explain how exhausted or unwell you feel, people respond with, "Well, you look great!" It may be well-intentioned, but it can come across as dismissive. Don't get me wrong, I believe the majority of people mean well.
Cancer-related fatigue is in a whole different league from the usual tiredness people experience. Being told, "That's just getting older," as though it's inevitable, is a real frustration. It's like I've acquired a whole new illness with no medication to fix it.

In fact, one of the more complex parts of cancer is the recovery stage, when surgery and treatment are behind you. The emotional toll is huge as you try to process everything. Again, this is invisible. The fear of recurrence weighs on you, as does the trauma that you have literally fought to stay alive. This doesn't leave you.

Words Can Sting
From chatting with breast cancer friends, I've found we collectively cringe at phrases like "Be positive" or "You have to be positive." While the intent might be good, it can come across as dismissive of the complexity of what we're going through. There's also the sympathetic head tilt or those well-meaning but detached reassurances like, "You'll be okay." When you live with the persistent knowledge that no one—not even your oncologist—can promise that, such words can feel empty.

Another friend was told, "You'll fly through it," when she was about to start chemotherapy. This was from someone who had been through treatment. So when she didn't "fly through it", she was shocked. Again, most people have the best intentions, but clearly, honesty would have been more helpful.

For me, one moment still stands out. I confided in someone I'm close to about feeling unsupported in some areas, only to hear, "When did you get so needy?" At the time, those words hurt.

Now, I smile because, often, comments like these come more from the speaker's own outlook than from an understanding of your situation.

Mental Health Matters
Since my diagnosis, I've really seen how mental health is as critical as physical health. I coped better with the gruelling effects of my treatment when my mental well-being was okay.

Throughout my illness, The Solas Centre, Waterford, was a haven for me. Whether I was dropping in for reflexology, attending a wellbeing workshop, or just grabbing a post-appointment coffee, I was always looked after and welcomed.

Outside of this, other ways I tried to support myself were through writing poetry, getting Reiki, spending time with loved ones and friends, and swimming at The Guillamene, Tramore, Co. Waterford, with the legends that frequent there. I've been called a "social butterfly" by some friends over the years, and they weren't wrong! There's nothing I enjoy more than sitting with friends at Molly's cafe in Tramore, or up having tea in the swim club cabin with fellow sea-lovers on any given day.

Dr. Jennifer Kilkus, Principal Specialist Psychologist at University Hospital Waterford, has kindly given her time and support to me throughout my cancer journey. Jennifer specialises in counselling oncology patients, so I thought, who better to talk to about some dos and don'ts when it comes to supporting someone with cancer.

What Not to Do
Jennifer explains that people often fall into certain categories when they don't know what to say. "Sometimes they make comments out of ignorance—they don't truly understand the experience—or they're not reflective enough to consider how their words might affect someone," she says. Relying on clichés or blurting out the first thought that comes to mind often results in words that unintentionally cause pain.

Here are some useful tips Jennifer highlighted:

- **Don't share upsetting cancer stories**
  Ever since my diagnosis, I've had people tell me about others who died from breast cancer. Then they suddenly stop, awkwardly realising how unhelpful it is. Jennifer sums it up perfectly: "If you find yourself sharing a story about someone you knew with cancer, and it ends with them dying, stop talking."

- **Don't blame or shame**
  Avoid asking questions about smoking, drinking, or other lifestyle behaviours when someone tells you they have cancer. These conversations can make a person feel as though they're to blame for their illness.

- **Don't compare tiredness**
  Saying you're tired too when someone mentions cancer-related fatigue reveals a lack of understanding. The exhaustion that comes with cancer is profound, not comparable to regular tiredness.

- **Avoid empty platitudes**
  Phrases like "You're so brave," "You're so strong," or "You'll be back to normal soon," while well-meaning, can feel trite and dismissive of the individual's pain and reality.

What You Can Do
Jennifer suggests a simple but effective approach to supporting someone with cancer—active listening. "This is rare," she says. "Most people listen to respond; they're just waiting for their turn to talk. Instead, focus on truly

listening to the other person's experience."

Here are some practical tips for being supportive:

- **Ask before offering advice**
  Before sharing any input, confirm whether it's wanted.

- **Show genuine care**
  Demonstrate curiosity about the person's experience in a respectful way.

- **Bring empathy into every interaction**
  Sometimes, listening without judgment or interruption can have a greater impact than anything else.

The Power of Connection
Supporting someone with cancer isn't about saying the perfect thing—it's about showing you care through thoughtful, empathetic actions and words. Being there and really listening can make a world of difference.

Poems

Bird
I'm a different bird now in every way
The flights I could take at my fancy
Now replaced with a plight of hospital appointments and treatment
Instead of a full head of messy feathers
My scalp is revealed and bare
Locks once thick and abundant
Now, a shadow of baby spikes protrudes from my head

If I beat my wings
They may take me to Tramore
Almost the furthest place I can venture to
When my body can get me there
It's a very different species I am now
Both inside and out
For sure, I'm a bird of a different kind

Migration
A large flock of birds migrate to somewhere distant
This seasonal movement away from a place that no longer provides
My breasts tried to kill me
They also no longer provide any good

The birds fly onwards
Their movement forward coincides with the fall of the leaves
The changing colours of the boggy landscape
It brings to mind my own migration from my previous life to where I am now
How far I've come and how far I must go

A migration from health to illness
Working life to not working
Love given to a new love, to being left alone
Years of swims to almost a year of none
Healthy breasts versus artificial replacements
Last but not least, long, thick hair to a shiny scalp
Shifting gears so many times

You feel like you've been taken apart, broken and put back together
Redesigned against your will
Chemo is like winter
Dark, empty and hard
And now I am here
A new normal

Farewell Old Me

To all the swims I did before
In a few days, there'll be no more
Beach, pier, Newtown and Guillamene
Take a bow 'cos ye served me well
On Thursday, I'll be entering my own hell

Say what you like, but 'tis only me who will still endure this gruelling journey
Friends and family at my side
Would like me to take this one in my stride
But I promise ye not I will, 'cos I've already been through the mill

Tramore and friends, I'll miss you
Even though you are all only a drive away
I'm counting on ye to have my back when I need you during the day
I know it's a lot to ask, but I hold you all in such esteem
Now I'd really love all this to be over so I can wake up from this bad dream

Swimming will be back for sure in time again
I promise I won't forget how good you've all been
Now onto what's next

What Would I Tell Her?
I wish I could return to the old me
What would I say to her?

I'd tell her if only you knew what's ahead
If she knew what was to be held over her
How, in a few moments, everything would change
Shards of glass would fall slowly towards you
Like slow motion, pieces covering your face

I'd tell you that what you would face would surpass all the other wars waged upon you over the years
So much grief, loss, loves lost and more
This is going to be different
This one would inherently show one's true fabric
How you'd deal with all the facets of this illness would cement who you are
Who you become
How you lived your life before may not resemble how you live now

Only you know the vastness of extent of the change and hardship inflicted on you
You patiently claw your way through the hell
And when it's over
You'll rise and dust off the dirt

While there will be more tears, coupled with worry and fear
You won't hang up your coat just yet

It's not your time
You have too much life to live
So much love to give

Kindness
Your smile when you see me
My face and your face light up
Don't think for a second that that isn't enough

You see, I'm on the other side now
I won't ever be going back
Your kindness matters a lot

If all you do when you see me is say a few friendly words
Or, spoil me with gifts here and there
Your kindness is bigger than anything else you do
The warm welcome, the laughs, the jokes

Keep smiling because it's enough

Meet The Follicles
I didn't know that after I shaved my head
Within days, I'd look like the 'Little Britain' guy in my bed
The locks were gone, and on the sheets, it was clear
I was lying in my own follicles right up to my ear

In the days before, once the trauma of losing my hair had happened
I got in the shower, water hitting my naked scalp felt quite mishappen
For the first time in days, I was almost scared of the droplets tumbling over my head
I felt so exposed to the world
I just wanted my bed

I called myself 'Harriet Dumpty' to my child
So as to appease her worried little mind
At nine years old, it was a lot to see
Her Mammy looking like an alien from that old show 'V'
It wasn't far from the truth

No hairdryer, no brushing anymore
Just a bit of cream on my head to show me some care
Oh, how shocking it was to see my reflection with no hair

Today, my hair is back, and I embrace my new follicles

I'm so grateful they're there
I'm less alien, no longer 'Little Britain'
I see my new hair as a way to define me
I touch it, play with it and essentially love it
It was a chapter in my life, I kid you not, laden with strife
A heavy burden I didn't ask for

But it's back, I'm still here and somewhat kicking each day in the ass

I leave with you this:
'Life is a gift. Go out there, search for the roses, take stock of all you have, and remember to lie in the grass.'

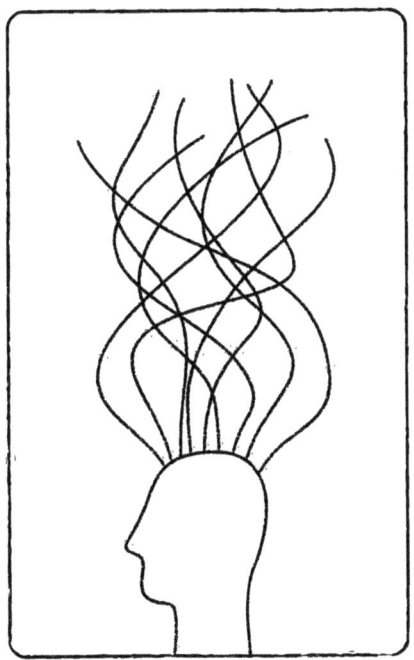

Cancer Rap
I'm not really in the mood to write
I feel like I'm living some 'lite' version of my life
This sucks, this is shit, I'm so sick of it
What's next for me?
When will this Cancer set me free?

The daily grind, so much left behind
Now my life revolves around what's barely mine
The sense of control is so minimal
This illness is so criminal
Would somebody come and make it better, so I can enjoy looking great in my favourite sweater

There is so much inside that wants to come out
Maybe a huge scream, maybe a shout
It's so hard to look at everybody else getting on with their lives
When all I want to do is be able to join and take what's mine

I love myself, I really do
I love everyone good to me, that includes you
I'm so sad for me, a personality that loves to live
C'mon, Cancer, when are you gonna give

The uncertainty, the fear, here I am, almost a year
I tell you this, I tell you true
I hope this never happens to you
The loneliness of being sick

Go away, Cancer, you're such a prick

Get Out Of My Way
The fatigue is unreal
This tiredness I feel
Day in, day out
Months pass, I'm wiped out

The walk I did the day before
I knew the cost would come knocking on my door
Heavy legs, groggy head
All I can think of is my comfy bed

This push in me to go forward
Live my day through people, and connection always wins
I'm too determined not to let Cancer get in my way
Though it's always there, hovering over my head
I promise myself I won't give in to my bed

I know myself that even with more rest
The fatigue will remain like a stubborn little pest
So off I go to get some air
I'll go for my walk, put on my make-up and style my hair
I'll show myself how much I can do
Then, come evening
I'll collapse on the chair

Feet up now, totally floored
But yippee, I did it
I got through the day

I tell you my friends
I wouldn't have it any other way

All The Right Things
Love your body
Feed it well
Drink enough water
Not too much alcohol
An active life
A nourished mind
Do all this and you'll be fine

Guidelines to keep you healthy
You follow them to the tee
When a bomb lands
You think, 'How can this be me?'

Bright eyes
Strong body
The picture of health
Cancer doesn't discriminate
It has a speed, a stealth

The ghostly ghoul strikes
You wake up one day
A body once loved becomes the enemy
Trust is overcome by betrayal
Scars, bumps, the lot
All along, was it part of the plot?

How long had it been growing
Before I felt it showing
It never feels over

I keep on going

A Bath Too Far
Bath poured, slip in
Hot enough, OK to go
Bare skin touches water
Feels like just before

Struck like a bolt of thunder
Head to toe
A massive sense of betrayal engulfs me
I'm devoured, swallowed whole
Confrontation too much
The clash of cover versus contents

Hot feet, soaped body
Almost all looks familiar
Trust gone, steam rising
Self-care, attempted self-love
Clean, defeated
Legs upright
A sense of hurriedness
prevails

A bath too far
Showed too much
The reveal
What lies beneath

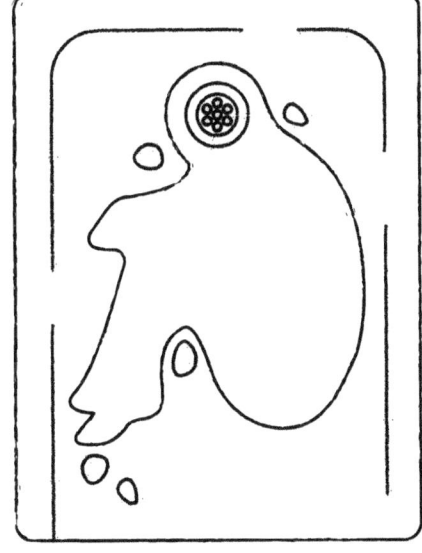

The Shadow
I see the reflection on my wall
This grand shadow stands tall
It clouds my head, intrudes on my day
By night, it hovers, lingers
It will do anything to find a way

Distraction prevails, but just for a bit
Slowly, it creeps in, working hard to be heard
Positive mindset and attitude reign
But soon again, the shadow toils away for my attention

This dark grafter looms over me now
It knows when to pounce
Its goal is to take me, it's coming for me
The darkness will try all consume me, envelope my body
It feeds on what I know
Which sometimes goes against me

In all of this, the shadow doesn't know everything
Night comes, the lights go off
Both reflection and shadow vanish
Just like that, gone

As I close my eyes, I know tomorrow will bring light and dark
New reflections, new shadow shapes and still

Life goes on

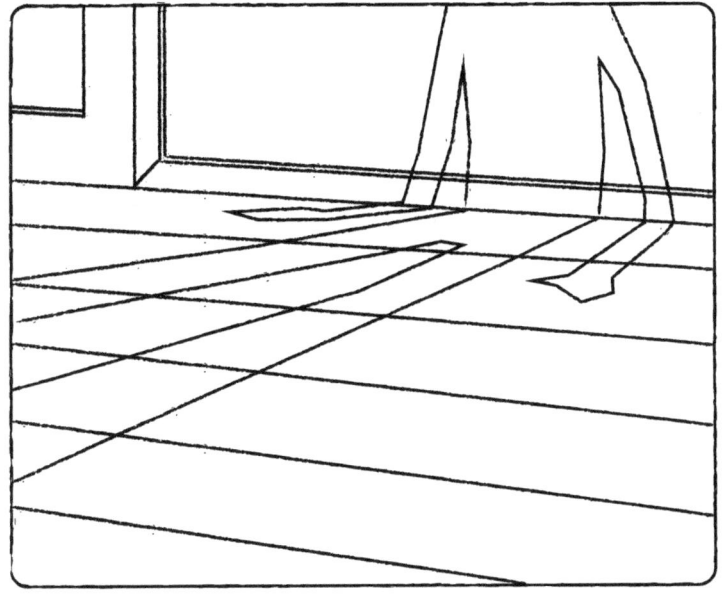

Altar of Aslan
I stand tall on top of this altar of stone
The power I feel looking out across the valley
I blink as the sun hits my face
The orange burning light beaming upon me

Everything is still, I summon his power
The strength of a lion, weighty paws, a proud head
A regal stance surveys the land
I want to reign like him
Reign mighty over my own life, my own land

The day closes in, the light fades
I walk away not as I came, but changed
Ready to enter a new phase

I'm here to serve the good and ally up with heroes
Those who face life's challenges yet seek peace, love and give
Live with the prowess and heart of a lion
Surround yourself with winners
All hail life

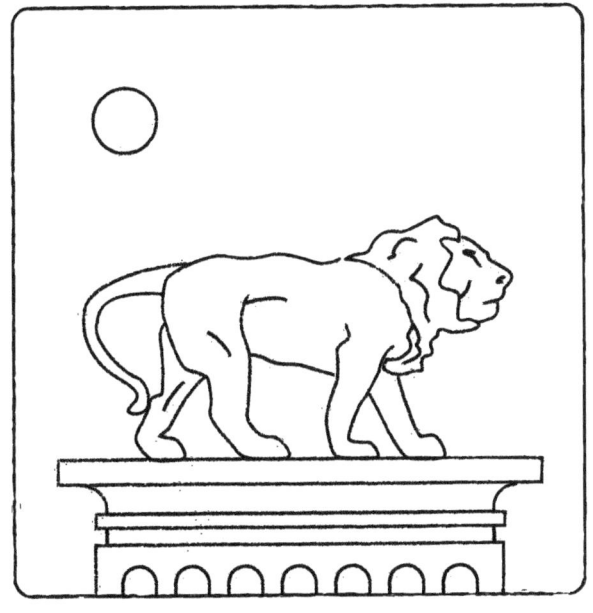

Peachy Ladies
To all the bras in my drawer
I do not need you anymore
Shocked, stunned, I know
But I have nowhere for you to go

White, pink, purple, red, yellow, blue
All the colours of the rainbow, black too
No discrimination, but my new ladies don't want you
The old ones 'moved on', so to speak
Under the care of SurgeonAir
They said their goodbyes the night before
6 hours later, I woke up with a new pair

It took some time for us to become familiar
There were many days when I longed for my old ones back
Months later, this pair has a new wardrobe, you see
They've a bit of a big head, just like me

Lace, cotton, silk, some with armour, some with pearl
You see, ladies, I've always been a material girl
I reach for my drawer and take my time
To see which one today
Will be on tomorrow's clothes line

It's a soft, peachy day, I think
I look at the ladies, and they give me a wink
Yes, that's the one, now off we go
We get in the car and follow the road that I know

We go for a spin out to Tramore
Where I love to take a dip in the sea
The ladies help keep me afloat
They bounce up and down, full of glee

Once I am dressed, I tell them to sit tight, not to move
They do as they're told, and all goes well
It almost makes me forget
How this pair and I met in hell

Almost a year later, we've bonded
We know each other better
On cold days, they're not as happy
But they do look good in my favourite sweater

In life, we don't always get a choice
It was very sad to say goodbye to my former pair
But it seems to be working out with these two
Time will tell, but for now, cheers ladies!

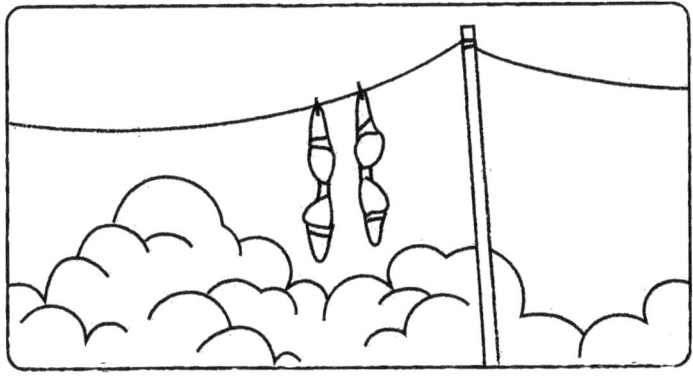

Come Sit With Me
You know I'm not well due to illness or grief
What do you say to me when I'm on my knees
My lowest, scariest time of my life
No words or text can suffice

You'd like to help make it better
Yet, all you worry about is what to say
I just want you to come sit with me

When all one can muster is to go from bedroom to kitchen
Body, energy and soul so low
All I want is for you to show

So come see my face
Know I'm suffering
You'll see I'm at my lowest place

Visits are everything
Texts don't always suffice
Food, chat, you by my side
All so welcome during my strife

People, love and kindness are what you need
So, don't worry about what to say
Just come sit with me

Share a cuppa, chat about anything
Then I'll know you care

When I'm better, I'll remember you came
You showed me you were there

Boom

My heart went boom that day in that room
Already dark, I filled it with my gloom
I won't forget that day in the Coombe
My stomach churns each time I'm upset
At this moment, I'm finding it hard to forget

Pain, feeling raw
Too often crap and grim
Wanting the day to come when I'll feel good again
I know this is a big crisis, you see
I'm hoping that in time, I'll be back to being me

On that day, my dream was taken
My head and heart went boom
That day, in that room

Cloud
The cloud lay its head down on the mountain
Its soft fluffiness enveloped the peak
A grey-blue hue bathed the surroundings
Trees bountiful beneath
A thick gorse bush encircled below
Roots, thick and strong, all along the bottom
As it went up, though, it got weaker at the top
The crowds looked on, staying hopeful
It looked insurmountable, but holding hands
They joined forces
Together we are strong

A Moment
Basking on a rock, the concrete's hot
The water lapping loudly below
Hands like ice, shivering myself back to warm
Flask at hand, the sun blasting my feet

A couple of seagulls swoop by
They land looking slightly cranky
Maybe they don't like the crowds
The sea is a little wavier than they'd like when landing

Others arrive to bathe and follow the same ritual
Some get up and go
It's a place to pass through and make yourself at home

The wind is picking up, the car calls
The cabin is closed, the gang have gone
Tomorrow, it will start all over again
It's time to go

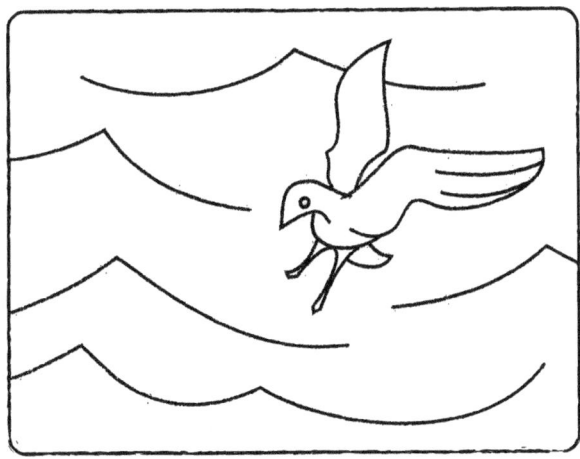

Immovable

The soil has been scraped back
A bigger mound of earth was there only yesterday
With the work, a few fingers and a bit of patting of the hands
The surface becomes more settled
The top is decorated
Adorned with flowers covering most of the ground
You glance around you and see the variety of efforts put in
Invested in making each one stand out
Like us, they're all different
But in the end, become the same
There's something about that ground that's so still and immovable
Just like her beneath

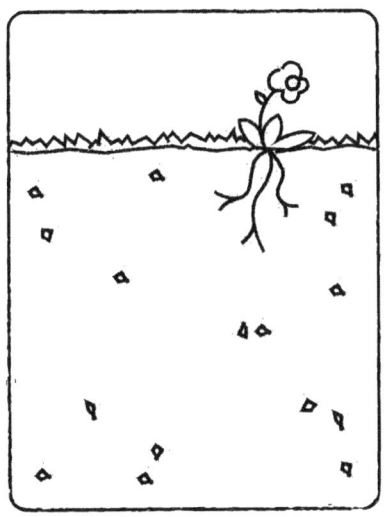

This Is Grief
My cheeks look shorn to the bone
Skin tight on my face, eyes sunken and sad
They hold a look that I'm not used to seeing staring back at me
This is grief

Fatigue, burnout, and disbelief take over the shock
The trauma of those hellish days we endured
She said, "I can't go", yet a few minutes later she was gone
Gasping for air, taking her last breaths in this world

Earlier on, we gowned up to go in and see her
We arrived at her sitting up
Beautiful blue eyes staring back at us, not knowing where she was
But we knew where we were

We were in the place where we would last see our mother alive
We cried helplessly around her bed
I rubbed her foot, my light touch jolted her
Even then, she still felt all that sensitivity in her foot
All the times she bribed us with a bag of Tayto to rub her feet
Looking back, sure, what did we know about how hard it must have been to raise seven children?

The priest entered the ICU

I remember saying to myself that this can't be it
He said, "Hello Ann, I was just passing by"
As he blessed her, my soul sank to a place so low

After that, more people came into the room
We watched the colour of her lips and face change
She took her last breath

Today, I carry that pain deep inside
The world isn't the same, and neither are we
Shaped by this forever

This is grief

She, The Sea

The sea forced me to look at myself
She forced me to let go
I dropped myself into the ocean
She would swell up to hold me, move me, catch me
Sometimes she would carry me to my destination
Be that cave, rock or pier
Other days, she shifts me left or right
You don't question her mode or her mood
She owes me nothing
She has nothing to fulfil
We give ourselves to her
She decides how we flow
Jump in, surrender
Trust and listen
You're in safe hands

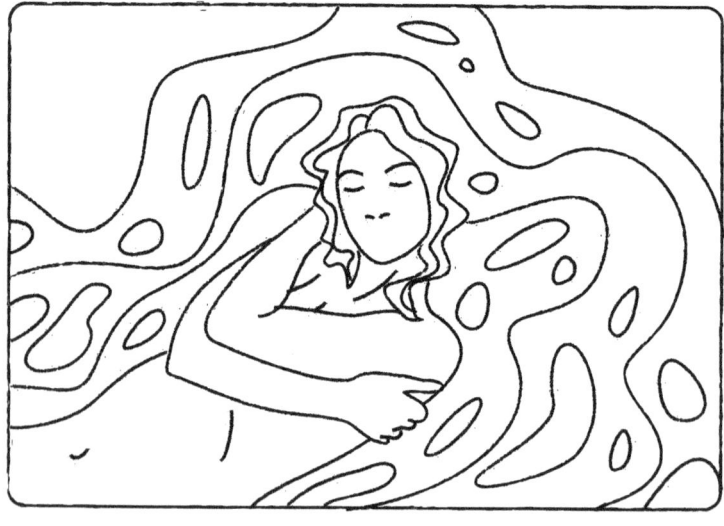

The Fox
There is something about the fox that's appealing
One could say it's quite concealing
It's time to take heed, time to go slow
Slow down
The chase is on

Often, it's one's fur that hides the deal
When the moment is right, the fur comes off
Slides off your shoulders
Drops to the floor
You drop to your knees and say 'Amen'

A New Kind of Boom
I'm back to Boom, but a new kind of Boom
This one's different
It's better than being in the Coombe
If I ever felt like an onion with layers on it, it's now
The layers have been peeled back
My head and heart under attack
Here we go again, never a dull moment, oh crapBut it's ok,
I'll get through this somehow
I always do
Bi-curious, whatever
Clearly, I can't wait forever
I need to keep it together
Or else, I could lose some very important people forever
And I don't want that
But hey, I have you to talk to, my baby and my cat
For now, I'll wear my straight mask
After all, it seems it's what I do best

That Mustard Chair
Firmly set in the sitting room
That mustard chair, so easy on the eye, holds a tale or two
Its arms, velvet and strong
Just like what I thought were her arms around me

Instead, I got what I didn't sign up for
Betrayal, fakeness and heartbreak
Two very different experiences going on in tandem
Her digressing away from me in secret
Me - ill, vulnerable and scared

Fooled by her words and her warm, funny facade
It was hard to see in something so short and sweet
A container, a host of deceit
I was robbed, stolen of what I thought was my future
Instead, I dodged a bullet

Too wholesome for she
Yet I still love this seat
It gives me some comfort
Takes the weight off my feet

Loss is hard, but real love
should win out
I wait patiently for the next
moment when our eyes connect
Only they won't be hers

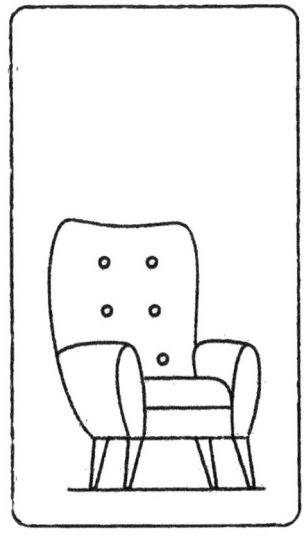

Flower

At dusk, your petals open and close just before dawn
This makes you special already
Strong, sweet and fragrant
Your form entices me closer
Your beauty draws me in
Under the moon, you stand out
I revel in your resplendence
Watching you blossom in front of my eyes
You in your place
Me, in mine
Our energies now entwined
The sun is rising
Your petals close in gently
I now know where you are
My Queen of the Night

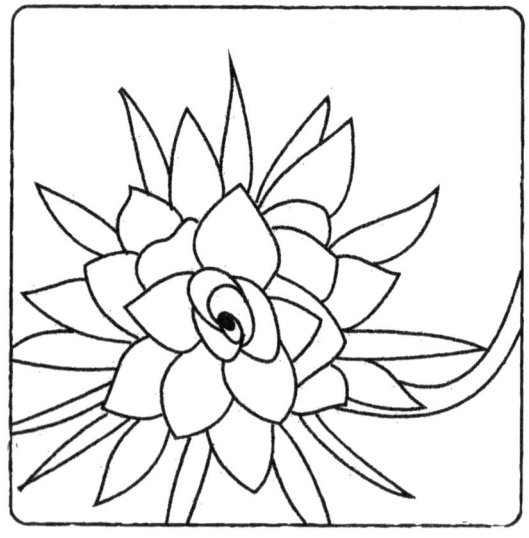

The Withering
Crinkled leaves, dry roots
Plant begs hydration
Stem strong but not for long
Silent screams flood the room
Unblock your ears
Tend to its needs
Take it out of the shadow
Open the blinds
Let the light in
See her suffering
Before she crumbles and withers

The Flame Has Gone Out
The flame has gone out
It's bloody sad, without a doubt
I think we both feel it's time to break out
What happened to us?

We used to be like soul mates, then best friends
Now we are like strangers
Not amused, no joke
The worst part, very little hope
Crash, bang, burn, baby
Another loud boom in our world

Where to next?
Who will take that first step?
It's getting close to crunch time
It's make or break
Harsh words were said
Me sleeping alone in my bed
Who knows what will happen next
Only time will tell
My mind is made up
I want to love again

Unoathed

You lay your hand over the book
Solemnly swear to tell the truth
You must perform when they say
You're under oath
There to speak only what is true

In those moments, a spell has been cast over you
An uncomfortable, heavy blanket of air weighs on you
Hovering over you all while your words flow
You address the inquisitors
It's crushing

You're conscious the whole way through
Yet the sense of time feels blurred
The clock keeps going forward
You feel nothing is going anywhere
Your lips are moving, articulating what you can
All the while conscious of being part of such a staged environment

Back and forward, it's eventually all done
Wrapped up under duress
In the days after, you experience the fallout
Pulling yourself together, waiting for the bad taste it left to go
The outcome will dictate the future

I hold onto what matters
I remain Unoathed

The Wolf
I met a wolf on my travels
I thought of this wolf only yesterday
I asked myself if it was still following me
Was it that that led me astray?

Face ashen, lying in the soil
Dirty, wet and cold, I lifted my head up
I could hardly see through the rain
The mist was thick, the forest quiet
I heard a scurry in the trees
Branches were breaking, and there was a squeal
My heart was racing

Breathing stifled by the noise, the unknown
He approached me
Eyes peering through the heavy air
Fur thick, grey and beautiful
My fur in shining armour

Relieved, I knew he could show me the way back out
He wouldn't hurt me
I slowly scraped myself off the ground
My legs staggered towards him
Something bad had happened to me, but there was a way out

He guided me, kept checking behind him to see if I was still there
I was

That night, he took me through the trees, the dark, the mist
Barefoot and wet, I got myself out
I saw the road
I had arrived
I didn't know where I was exactly, but I had got there

Today, I have the strength of that Wolf

Notes

Bird — p.17
Written after chemo in 2024, I felt so changed inside and out.

Migration — p. 18
Without a doubt, cancer takes you from the body and the life you knew to a new, scary, gruelling place. Like a migration of sorts, but not by choice. Seeing a flock of birds one day fly to somewhere distant, the image of migration stuck with me and inspired this piece.

Farewell Old Me — p. 19
This poem was extremely emotional for me. I wrote it the night before my surgery on June 26th. I recorded it and sent it to a special group of friends. I remember one of them ringing me in tears as they knew how hard this was for me. It still tugs at me and makes me feel raw when I see it. I knew my body would be changed forever the next day.

What Would I Tell Her? — p. 20
I wrote this a few months after my diagnosis. I felt sad for myself, someone who enjoyed life so much. So much was taken from me in an instant and I had to face this horrible journey.

Kindness — p. 21
After my surgery, once I started to get back on my feet (just in time for radiotherapy and more chemo…), I was able to go out and socialise again.

When friends saw me, I got such the warmest of smiles, hugs and reception and I was as happy to give the same back. All of the kindness I received meant more to me than ever. It really enhanced my appreciation of good people.

Meet The Follicles — p. 22
Well, this one of the most standout elements of my cancer experience. The trauma of losing my long, thick hair after my second chemo session was horrendous. It was as bad as being told I had a second cancer.

To this day, I still hold a lot of trauma about this part of my identity being taken from me. For me, it is a massive thing for a woman to go through in parallel to having a very awful chemotherapy experience.

Cancer Rap — p. 24
I wrote this piece out of sheer frustration on not being able to live my life the way 1 wanted and just suffering with it all. I felt like it would never get easier or normal again. Reality is, cancer changes you forever at a very deep level so it's hard to accept this. I longed not to be the sick one.

Get Out Of My Way — p. 25
I have had a very tough time with cancer-related fatigue and it really impacted my day to day quality of life. It is like an additional illness and unless you have experienced it, people don't seem to understand it.

Another element to cancer to endure.

Not everyone is affected the same way or as severe. It is something that I have pushed through so much so that I could enjoy my day but then always pay a price.

All The Right Things — p. 26
I've been a vegetarian most of my life, active, non-smoker and mid-40's. At 46, I get diagnosed with one of the rarer, more aggressive breast cancers that had already spread to some lymphnodes.

February 8, the news that I had cancer was just a nuclear bomb to my life and my being. I couldn't believe that it wasn't just a cyst and that it was one of the harder ones to treat.

And, most likely to recur...

Anyone in my shoes would ask themselves how the hell did this happen when I took care of myself all my life and lead a healthy lifestyle.

I tested positive for a Chek2 gene mutation which could have been the reason I got breast cancer. But then that leaves 60% other possible factors in my head. In the end, you have to move on from the 'why'.

A Bath Too Far — p. 27
One evening I got into the bath and looked down at my body.

This was in April 2025, well over a year after my diagnosis in February 2024.

My mood changed from enjoying the water, to suddenly feeling just so upset.

It was the fact that most of my body looked the same, minus my chest area and hair. I got freaked out by what could be lurking under the sameness. My skin looked healthy, all of me. I felt such a sense of betrayal by my own body. I couldn't get out of the bath quick enough.

The Shadow — p. 28
Fear of recurrence follows fairly quickly after treatment is completed. For me especially, my chemo was halted early before my surgery and also, a second round of chemo in October 2024 had to be stopped. The fact my body couldn't tolerate the chemo adds more worry to me than maybe if I had been able to complete the prescribed amount of cycles.

Keeping busy and filling your life with love, laughs and plenty of distraction really helps push it to the back of your mind.

Altar Of Aslan — p. 30
Early 2025, I was looking out across the valley in South Kilkenny at my daughter playing with her friend. The view

was amazing and the sun was going down, I looked down and realised I was standing on some sort of big slab of stone. It looked like an old altar and in that moment, I felt quite powerful. This felt special. All I wanted was to savour being alive and moving forward.

Peachy Ladies — p. 32
As I lay in my bed in April 2025 (I think), I saw a bra strap dangling from my drawer. It evoked feelings of sadness and longing for my own breasts, not numb, implants that I now have to get used to and still am a year later.

Breast cancer is so complex and affects mind, body and soul. I can no longer wear my old bras due to soreness and different shape. The bras are still in my drawer because I haven't emotionally gotten to the point where I have to look at them and throw them away. Not one person who has gone through a mastectomy has ever really opened up about this being a 'thing' for them.

I made light out of a very difficult subject here and it has helped somewhat in the acceptance of my new 'ladies'.

Come Sit With Me — p. 34
After my surgery in June 2024, it was a long summer of recovery before heading into radiotherapy and more chemo. I live in the countryside and couldn't drive for 6 weeks. The visitors who came to spend time with me really kept me going mentally, as the days were long and I was too weak to go far for a while. Company, generosity, and compassion were everything.

Boom — p. 35
This is a very personal, sad poem for me when I had a miscarriage in 2014. I went to a lady in Dublin for Reiki and that night, I wrote my first ever poem about my loss and the darkness of that experience.

Cloud — p. 36
During COVID, I used to hike up Tory Hill, South Kilkenny a few times a week. It was covered in trees and gorse bush. It inspired me to write this little poem about as daunting as something looks, joining forces we are stronger together.

A Moment — p. 37
The day after my sister's wedding I was longing for a swim and some alone time so off I went to the Guillamene, Tramore, Co. Waterford for a dip.

I sat under the wall where people get changed and there was nothing between me and sea. I observed the seagulls, the people come and go while sipping on my tea. It was a very peaceful, reflective moment.

Immovable — p. 38
My mother, Anne, died at 74 years of age in November 2022. It wasn't cancer related and it hit me and my family very hard. On her first anniversary, my father and brother went to her grave to prepare it for the headstone. It was a very difficult few days, like we were losing her all over again. It was overwhelmingly sad.

This is Grief — p. 40
This piece describes the passing of my 74-year-old mother back in November 2022.

She, The Sea — p. 42
This short poem is all about my love of the sea and what my experience is like when I'm immersed in the water.

It's one of my favourite things to do and I find it very healing while recovering from cancer.

That Mustard Chair — p. 45
I'll say very little about this piece except that the person that I thought I had by my side during cancer and before my surgery just up and went one night. I was left alone to face the rest.

They told me to hold on to their beloved mustard chair as it added colour to my sitting room... I could use very colourful language here but this is a poetry book. It left me broken hearted and very vulnerable. A highly unpleasant experience.

Flower — p. 46
This poem feels magical and mystical to me. I love the idea of a flower blooming at night, but gone the next morning.

About Ciara
Born in Waterford and raised in Co. Kilkenny, Ciara Foskin, aged 47, was diagnosed with a rare form of breast cancer in February 2024.

Mother to 11 year old Saibh, Ciara has always had a zest for life and loves nothing more than to be in the sea with her friends. The cancer diagnosis hit hard and through creative writing, Ciara found writing poetry as a way to express the emotional and physical side of cancer.

She hopes her words will help others going through illness and grief.

Acknowledgements

To my daughter Saibh, aged 11, who has been a little trouper to her mammy throughout cancer.

A big thank you to Emer Phelan, a true friend and support in every way, who has helped carry me through the past 12 months post-surgery. Her loyalty to me and my daughter has been so appreciated and needed.

Thanks to Dave Comiskey, who has been amazing to work with on my first poetry book.

To Dr. Jennifer Kilkus, Onco-Psychologist, for being a huge emotional support to me since my diagnosis and for her contribution to my book.

To the Solas Centre, Waterford, and the Marie Keating Foundation, who have brought comfort to my life.

A very important thank you to all the nurses and doctors at University Hospital Waterford and UPMC Whitfield for taking care of me during my illness.

To all my wonderful friends and family, far and near, love you lots - thank you.

Finally, a special call out to The Guillamene and Newtown Cove swim club, Tramore, Co. Waterford, who have been there for me throughout a gruelling 2024. They continue to bring sunshine, laughs, and heart-warming moments to my life. You are my tribe.

www.ingramcontent.com/pod-product-compliance
Lightning Source LLC
Chambersburg PA
CBHW061235070526
44584CB00030B/4127